GET SLIM NOW RECIPES

An Illustrated Cookbook of Guiltless Dish Ideas!

Table of Contents

Introduction

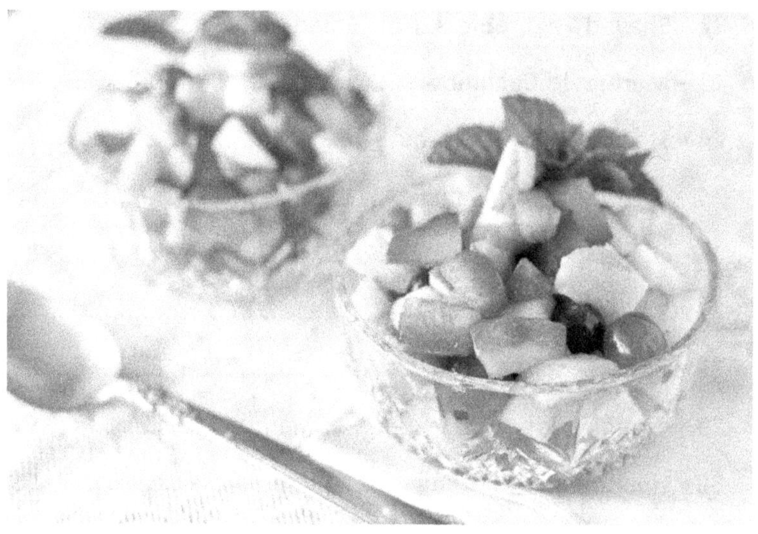

Some time ago, recently or farther back, did you decide to eat healthier to maintain a slim body? Or to reveal the slim figure you used to have?

You'll realize soon that you need to eat the right foods if you want to slim down or stay slim. Even if you eat salads for lunch at fast-food restaurants, they aren't much healthier than the burgers and fries they sell. They make you feel heavy and bloated and you'll feel your energy waning long before the end of your shift.

The secret? You need to make your slim meals at home, where you'll control ingredients and portions, and save money over eating out, too.

At first, doing your meals at home will save money and boost energy. And that would be enough, but there's more. After a few weeks, you'll be seeing weight loss. It's almost a surprise, because you won't feel that you've been denying yourself anything.

You can't see how the ingredients are prepared when you eat out. In your kitchen, you have complete control. You'll be making most recipes without butter or corn syrup, and you'll go easy on the salad dressing. Don't buy anything that might tempt you at home. Remove that option to more easily achieve or maintain a slim figure.

When you take your meals into your own hands, making them in your own kitchen, it's an empowering thing. All your choices are healthy. Turn the page, let's start cooking healthy...

You can enjoy tasty breakfasts and still get slim or keep slim. Here are a few of the best recipes...

1 – Overnight Chocolate & Chia Oats

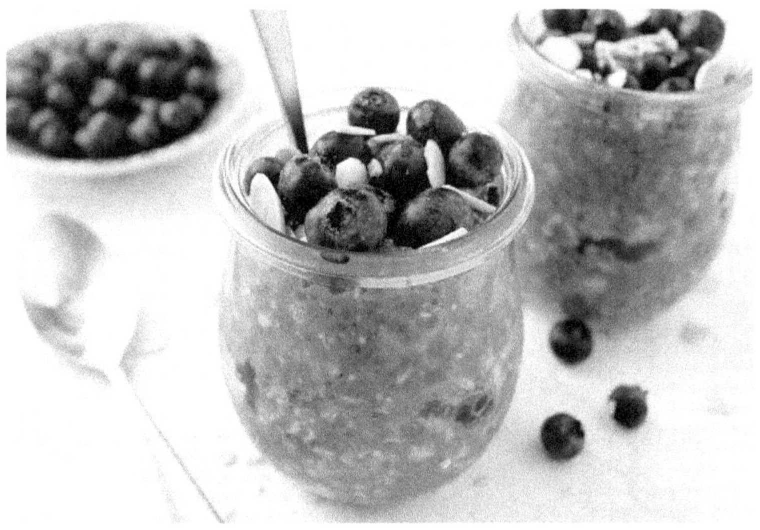

There's nothing like starting your day off with chocolate, right? And this recipe is STILL healthy! All you need is chia seeds, rolled oats, almond milk, syrup and yogurt.

Makes 2 Servings

Cooking + Prep Time: 15 minutes

Ingredients:

- 1 cup of oats, rolled
- 3 tbsp. of powdered cocoa
- 1 tbsp. of chia seeds

- 1/4 cup of yogurt, Greek

- A pinch of kosher salt

- 1 cup of unsweetened almond milk, low fat

- 2 tbsp. of syrup, maple

- 1 tsp. of vanilla extract, pure

Instructions:

1. Mix the dry ingredients together in medium bowl.

2. Add the wet ingredients to the mixture and combine well.

3. Cover and place in fridge for two hours at a minimum. Overnight is even better.

4. Top with the yogurt and fresh, sliced strawberries. Serve cold.

Nutrition Information

Serving Size: 1/2 cup

Calories: 281

Sugar: 15 grams

Fat: 7 grams

Carbohydrates: 48 grams

Fiber: 9 grams

Protein: 11 grams

2 – Veggie Breakfast Quiche

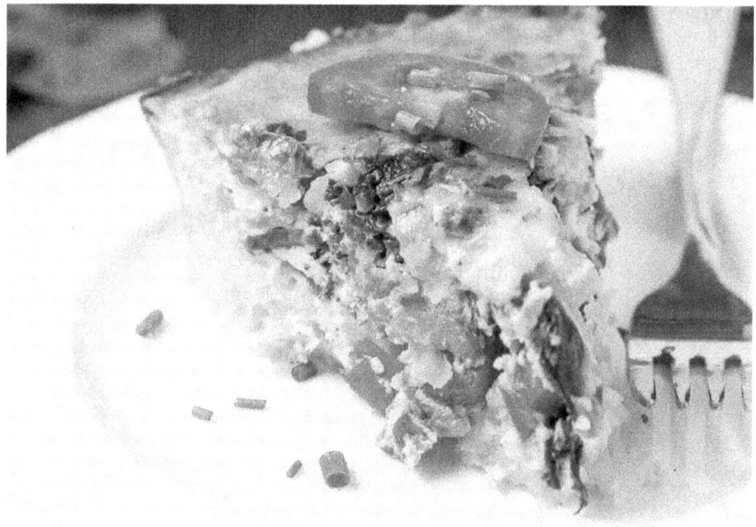

This quiche has no crust, so it is much lower in calories than traditional quiches. It's a low carb option, bursting with flavor from mushrooms, bell peppers and kale.

Makes 8 Servings

Cooking + Prep Time: 1 hour

Ingredients:

- 2 minced garlic cloves
- 2 tbsp. of oil, olive
- 3 sliced green onions

- 1/2 cup of diced bell peppers

- 2 cups of sliced mushrooms, button

- 3 cups of chopped kale

- 12 eggs, large

- 1/2 cup of 1% milk

- 1/2 tsp. of salt, kosher

- 1/4 tsp. of pepper, ground

- 1/2 tsp. of thyme, fresh

- 1 cup of shredded cheese, Asiago

Instructions:

1. Preheat the oven to 350F. Prepare 10-inch x 12-inch casserole dish with non-stick spray and set it aside.

2. Heat oil on med. in large sized skillet. Add bell peppers, garlic and green onions. Sauté them till a bit tender, usually about two to three minutes.

3. Add the mushrooms and sauté till somewhat tender, two minutes or so.

4. Fold in the kale and sauté till it wilts, or about one minute.

5. Remove pan from the heat. Pour into casserole dish prepared above.

6. Whisk milk, eggs, thyme, kosher salt and ground pepper in large sized bowl. Pour mixture over the vegetables in casserole dish. Add cheese on top.

7. Leave uncovered and bake for 35 to 45 minutes, till eggs have set.

8. Remove dish from the oven and serve while warm.

Nutrition Information

Serving size: 8 ounces

Calories: 210

Fat: 13 grams

Saturated Fat: 4 grams

Sodium 457 milligrams

Carbohydrates 5 grams

Sugar 2 grams

Protein 15 grams

3 – Blueberry Yogurt & Oatmeal Pancakes

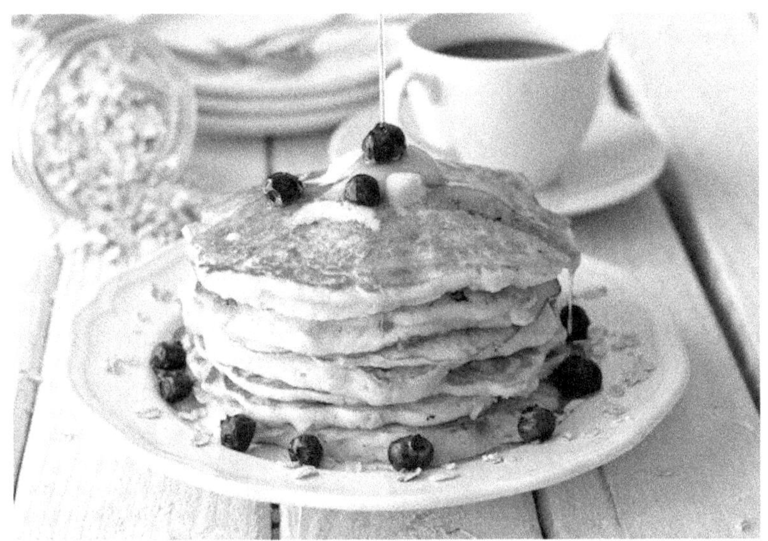

These pancakes are so easy to make. Just toss the ingredients in your food processor, process and then you're ready to pour and cook for a slim-friendly breakfast.

Makes 2 Servings

Cooking + Prep Time: 15 minutes

Ingredients:

- 1/2 cup of oats, rolled, gluten-free
- 1/2 tsp. of baking powder

- 1 x 5 & 1/4-ounce yogurt, vanilla bean
- 1/2 of a medium banana, ripe
- 1 egg, large
- 1/2 tsp. of vanilla, pure
- 1/3 cup of frozen or fresh blueberries + extra to serve

Instructions:

1. Place all the ingredients with the exception of the blueberries into food processor. Process till you have a smooth consistency. Set the batter aside and allow it to thicken for several minutes.

2. Coat large skillet lightly with cooking spray. Heat on med-low. Drop the batter 1/4 cup at a time into the skillet. Add a few blueberries.

3. Cook pancakes till they have bubbles on the top. Flip the cakes. Cook till golden brown on second side.

4. Wipe the skillet till it's clean. Spray again with non-stick spray and make pancakes from remining batter. Serve warm with maple syrup.

Nutrition Information

Serving size: 2 small pancakes

Calories: 210

Fat: 3.8 grams

Carbohydrates: 29.4 grams

Sugar: 12.8 grams

Fiber: 3.3 grams

Protein: 13.6 grams

4 – Beans & Greens with Poached Eggs

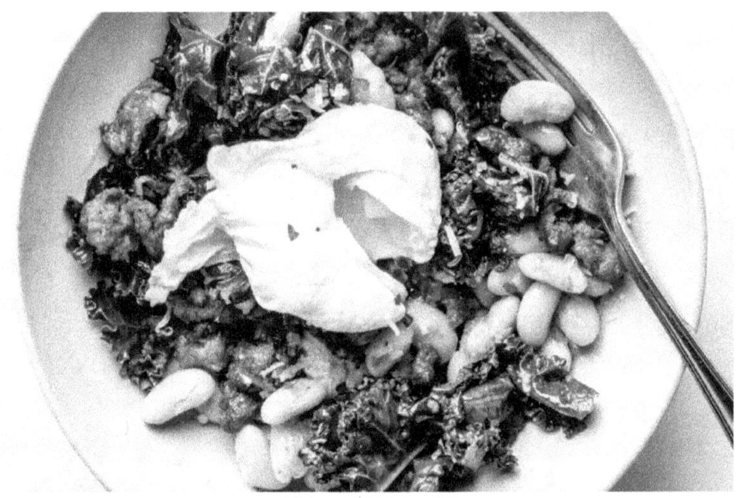

You may have cans of these white beans in your pantry and not even remember them. Dig them out and use them for this beans and greens hash – it's great!

Makes 4 Servings

Cooking + Prep Time: 25 minutes

Ingredients:

- 1 x 15-oz. can of rinsed, drained cannellini beans
- 3 tbsp. of oil, olive
- 1 tsp. of salt, kosher

- 1 tsp. of za'atar spice blend

- 1 bunch of de-stemmed, sliced Swiss chard

- 2 minced garlic cloves

- 1/4 tsp. of pepper flakes, red + extra to serve

- 1 tbsp. of lemon juice, fresh-squeezed

- 4 poached eggs, large

Instructions:

1. Heat 2 tbsp. of oil in large fry pan on med-high till it shimmers.

2. Add beans and spread them evenly on bottom of pan. Leave alone while they cook till beans have browned lightly on underside, or two to four minutes.

3. Add 1/2 tsp. of salt & 1 tsp. of za'atar spice blend. Combine by stirring. Spread beans out evenly again. Stir as needed while cooking till golden brown in color with blisters on each side.

4. Add last 1 tbsp. of oil to pan. Add chard, last 1/2 tsp. of salt & last tsp. of za'atar. Add pepper flakes and garlic. Stir occasionally while cooking till chard wilts, or three to five minutes.

5. Remove pan from heat. Add lemon juice. Toss and combine well. Divide greens and beans into four individual bowls. Top them with one poached egg each and red pepper flakes. Serve while warm.

Nutrition Information

Serving size: 1/4 of recipe ingredients (1 small plate)

Calories: 298

Fat: 15 & 1/2 grams

Saturated Fat: 3 grams

Carbohydrates: 26 & 1/2 grams

Fiber: 6 & 1/2 grams

Sugar: 1 & 1/2 gram

Protein: 15 & 1/2 grams

Sodium: 565 milligrams

5 – Sweet Potato & Almond Butter Breakfast

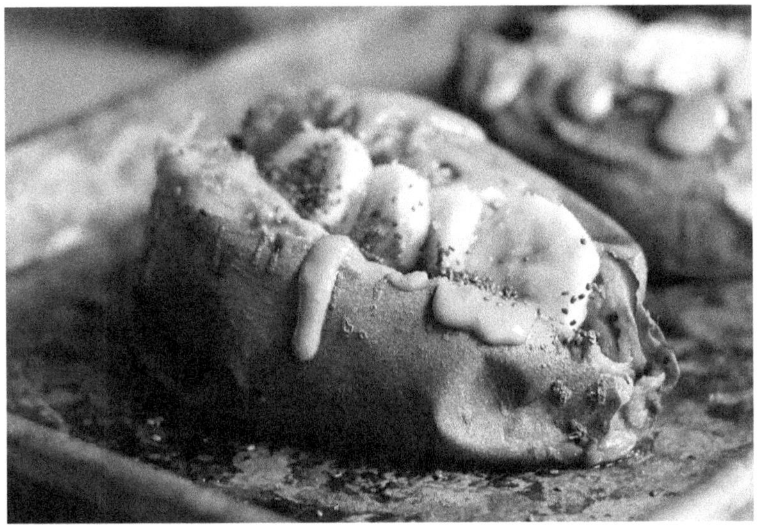

This is an easy to make breakfast with a taste like dessert. You'd never know it will help to keep you slim. It includes sweet potatoes, almond butter and sliced bananas to create such a wonderful treat.

Makes 2 Servings

Cooking + Prep Time: 55 minutes

Ingredients:

- 2 washed sweet potatoes, medium
- 2 tbsp. of almond butter, natural
- 1 sliced banana
- 2 tsp. of chia seeds
- Cinnamon, ground
- Salt, sea

Instructions:

1. Preheat the oven to 375F. Line medium cookie sheet with baking paper.

2. Poke some holes in sweet potatoes with fork. Place on the prepared cookie sheet. Roast them for 45 minutes to one hour, till fork-tender.

3. Remove sweet potatoes from the oven. Let them cool for five to 10 minutes.

4. Split them open and sprinkle a little salt inside. Drizzle 1 tbsp. almond butter and 1 tsp. of chia seeds and sliced bananas. Sprinkle cinnamon into each. Serve promptly.

Nutrition Information

Serving size: 1 sweet potato, stuffed

Calories: 282

Fat: 9.4 grams

Saturated fat: 1 gram

Carbohydrates: 44.7 grams

Sugar: 19.1 grams

Fiber: 9.4 grams

Protein: 7.7 grams

There is no shortage of healthy dishes that help you stay slim, from lunch and supper to side dishes and appetizers. Here are some of the best…

6 – Steak & Watermelon Salad

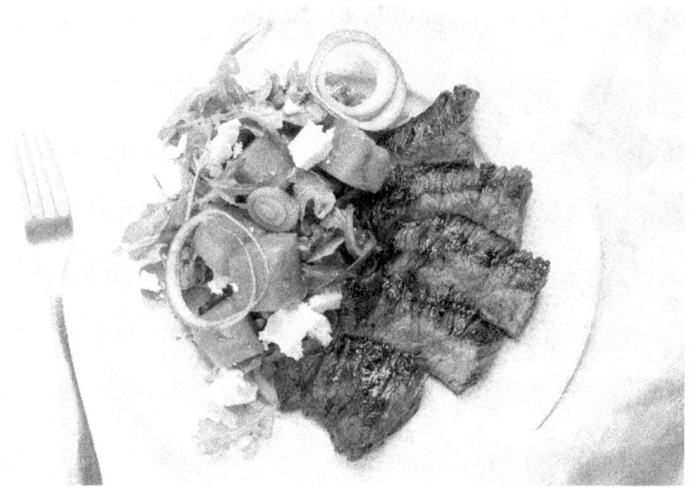

In this recipe, you'll grill steak and watermelon and serve them with a colorful, bright salad. It's a perfect salad for those long summer days.

Makes 4 Servings

Cooking + Prep Time: 35 minutes

Ingredients:

- 4 x 1" thick sliced steaks, beef tenderloin
- 1 tsp. of coriander, ground
- 1 tsp. of cumin, ground
- 2 slices of 1" thick watermelon, seedless

- Salt, kosher

- Pepper, ground

- 8 cups of spinach or arugula leaves

- 1 cup of cherry tomatoes, halved

- 1/4 cup of Italian or balsamic dressing, reduced fat

- 1/2 cup of red onion, sliced thinly

- 1/4 cup of feta cheese crumbles, reduced fat

Instructions:

1. Combine the cumin and coriander and evenly press in steaks.

2. Place the steaks in middle of grill over med. coals. Arrange the slices of watermelon around the steaks.

3. Cover grill and grill the steaks for 10-14 minutes on med. heat. Turn them occasionally.

4. Grill the watermelon for two to four minutes, turning once, till you can see grill marks on them.

5. Carve steaks in slices. Slice watermelon into wedges. Season both as desired.

6. Next, combine the dressing and arugula in a large sized bowl. Toss and coat greens with dressing.

7. Divide the arugula on four individual plates. Arrange the watermelon and steaks on the salad. Evenly top with cheese, tomatoes and onions. Serve.

Nutrition Information

Serving Size: 1 steak + 1 bowl watermelon & salad

Calories: 287

Fat: 10 grams

Cholesterol: 70 milligrams

Sodium: 335 milligrams

Carbohydrates: 25 grams

7 – Pumpkin & Garlic Soup

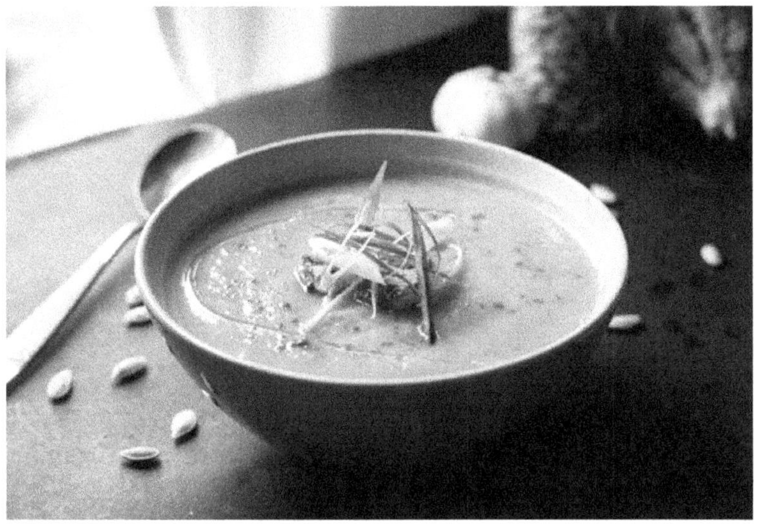

This lunch or dinner recipe is a cream-like and delicious soup that is often served in families' Thanksgiving dinners each year. It's a great way to stay slim without sacrificing flavor.

Makes 8 Servings

Cooking + Prep Time: 1 hour & 20 minutes

Ingredients:

- 6 cups of stock, chicken
- 1 & 1/2 tsp. of salt, kosher

- 4 cups of pureed pumpkin

- 1 tsp. of chopped parsley, fresh

- 1 cup of onion, chopped

- 1/2 tsp. of chopped thyme, fresh

- 1 minced garlic clove

- 1/2 cup of whipping cream, heavy

- 5 whole peppercorns, black

Instructions:

1. Heat the chicken stock, peppercorns, garlic, thyme, onion, pumpkin and salt. Bring to boil, then reduce the heat down to low. Simmer uncovered for 1/2 hour.

2. Puree soup in one-cup batches at a time in food processor.

3. Return soup to the pan. Bring back to boil. Reduce the heat down to low. Simmer uncovered for another 1/2 hour.

4. Add and stir cream. Pour soup in individual bowls. Use parsley to garnish. Serve.

Nutrition Information

Serving size: 1 bowl

Calories: 120

Fat: 6.5 grams

Carbohydrates: 13.8 grams

Protein: 2.9 grams

Cholesterol: 25 milligrams

Sodium: 1450 milligrams

8 – Scrambled Egg & Bean Tacos

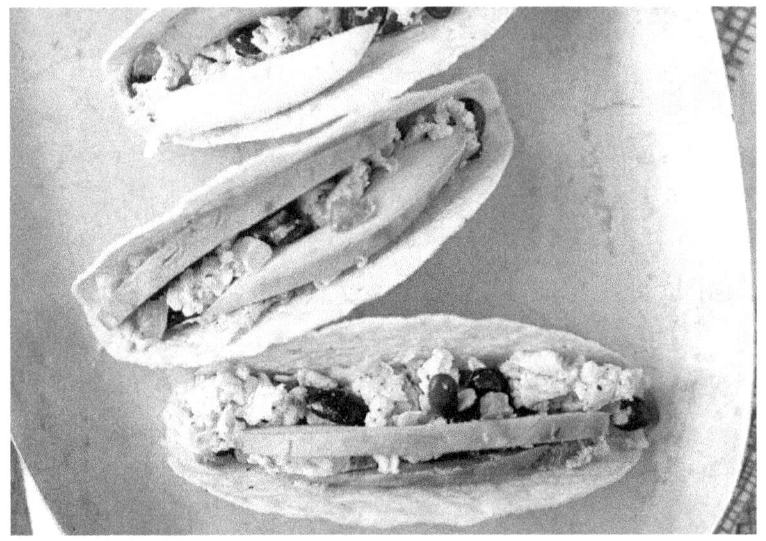

This recipe is like having breakfast for your dinner. These bean and egg tacos are full of healthy protein, and you'll feel full till it's time to hit the bed.

Makes 4 Servings

Cooking + Prep Time: 20 minutes

Ingredients:

- 1 x 15-ounce can of rinsed beans, black

- 2 tbsp. of oil, olive

- 1/2 tsp. cumin seeds

- 1 chopped garlic clove
- Salt, kosher
- Pepper, ground
- 4 cups of spinach, baby
- 1 tbsp. of lemon juice, fresh
- 8 eggs, large
- 8 tortillas, corn

To serve:

- Cilantro, sour cream and queso fresco crumbles

Instructions:

1. Heat a tbsp. of oil in large-sized skillet over med. heat. Add garlic, beans and cumin.

2. Season using 1/8 tsp. of kosher salt & 1/8 tsp. of ground pepper. Cook till the garlic begins turning golden brown in color. Add the spinach.

3. Remove pan from heat. Toss till leaves have barely wilted. Add and stir lemon juice.

4. Whisk eggs, 1 tbsp. filtered water, 1/2 tsp. each kosher salt and ground pepper together in large sized bowl.

5. Heat last tbsp. of oil in small skillet over med. heat. Add the eggs. Stir while cooking every couple of seconds till done as you desire.

6. Char tortillas lightly over gas flame or under a broiler. Fill the tortillas with eggs and beans. Add cilantro, sour cream and queso fresco, if you like. Serve.

Nutrition Information

Serving size: 2 tacos

Calories: 455

Fat: 23 grams

Protein: 24 grams

Sodium: 780 milligrams

Carbohydrates: 44 grams

9 – Mushroom & Green Bean Medley

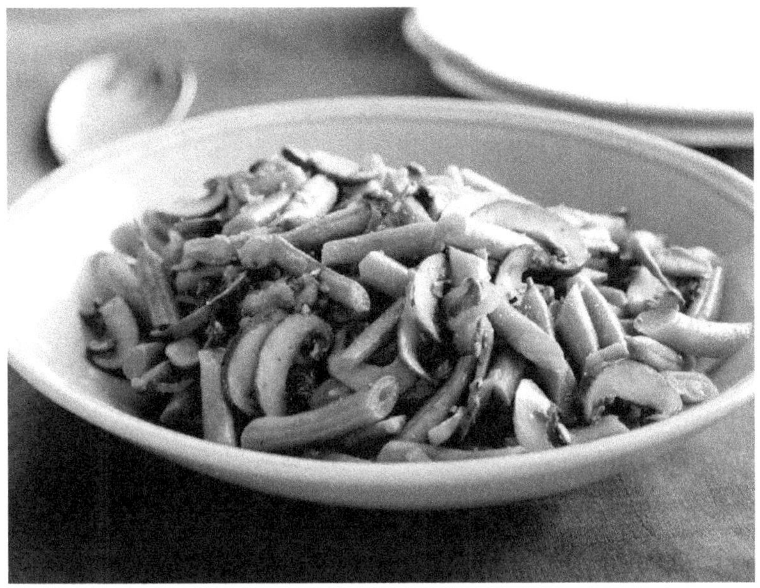

Green beans and mushrooms make this a great slimming veggie side dish. We serve it at many family parties and get-togethers, and we never have any leftovers.

Makes 6 Servings

Cooking + Prep Time: 40 minutes

Ingredients:

- 2 thick-cut carrots
- 1/2 lb. of 1"-length cut green beans, fresh

- 1/4 cup of butter, unsalted
- 1 sliced onion
- 1/2 lb. of sliced mushrooms, fresh
- 1 tsp. of salt, kosher
- 1/2 tsp. of salt, seasoned
- 1/4 tsp. of pepper, white
- 1/4 tsp. of garlic salt

Instructions:

1. Place carrots and green beans in one inch boiling water. Then cover the pan and cook till they are tender, yet still firm, and drain them.

2. Melt the butter in large sized skillet on med. heat. Sauté mushrooms and onions till nearly tender.

3. Reduce the heat and cover the pan. Simmer for three minutes. Add and stir carrots, beans, garlic salt, seasoned salt, kosher salt and white pepper.

4. Cover pan. Cook for about five minutes on med. heat. Serve.

Nutrition Information

Serving size: 1 small bowl or small plate

Calories: 110

Fat: 8 grams

Carbohydrates: 7.9 grams

Protein: 2 grams

Cholesterol: 22 milligrams

Sodium: 605 milligrams

10 – Farro & Honey Burrito Bowls

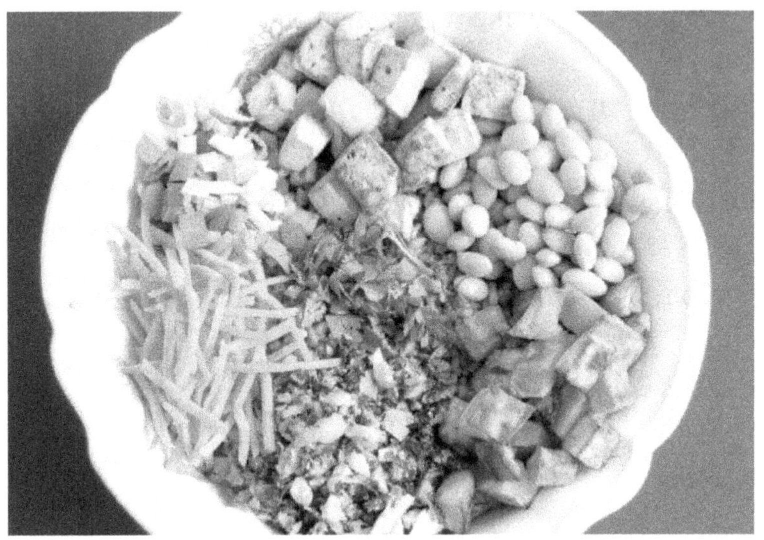

Here is a colorful, healthy-grain recipe that you can make ahead for lunch or dinner. The farro is simmered for less than half an hour, then drained, cooled and refrigerated. Then it's ready to go!

Makes 4 Servings

Cooking + Prep Time: 1/2 hour

Ingredients:

- 2 tbsp. of chopped cilantro, fresh
- 3 tbsp. of oil, olive

- 2 tbsp. of lime juice, fresh
- 2 tsp. of honey, pure
- 3/4 tsp. powdered ancho chili
- 3/4 tsp. of salt, kosher
- 1/2 tsp. of pepper, ground
- 2 cups of farro, cooked
- 2 cups of coarsely chopped vegetable mixture, grilled
- 1 x 15-ounce can of rinsed, drained black beans, unsalted
- 3 oz. of crumbled queso fresco
- 1 sliced avocado, medium
- Lime wedges, fresh

Instructions:

1. Combine the first seven ingredients together in medium-sized bowl and stir with whisk. Reserve 1 & 1/2 tbsp. of cilantro mixture. Add the farro to the rest of the cilantro mixture and toss to evenly coat.

2. Divide the chopped vegetables, farro mixture, cheese, avocado and beans into four shallow bowls. Drizzle with last cilantro mixture. Garnish with lime wedges. Serve.

Nutrition Information

Serving size: 2 cups

Calories: 461

Fat: 25 grams

Protein: 17 grams

Carbohydrates: 55 grams

Cholesterol: 16 milligrams

Sodium: 610 milligrams

Sugars: 8 grams

11 – Lentil Curry

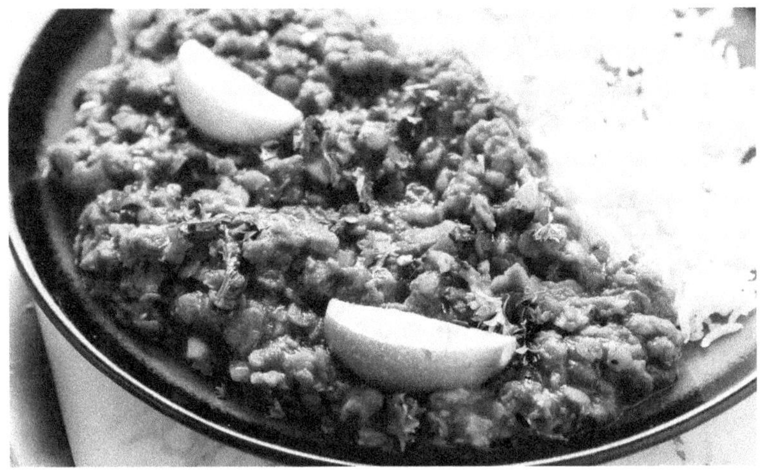

This hearty, rich lentil curry works well as an entrée, instead of a side dish like traditional Indian curries. The ingredient list is a bit long, but it's super easy to make and it works well for those trying to slim down.

Makes 8 Servings

Cooking + Prep Time: 45 minutes

Ingredients:

- 2 cups of lentils, red
- 1 diced onion, large
- 1 tbsp. of oil, vegetable

- 1 tsp. of cumin, ground

- 1 tsp. of turmeric, ground

- 1 tbsp. of curry powder

- 2 tbsp. of curry paste

- 1 tsp. of salt, kosher

- 1 tsp. of chili powder

- 1 tsp. of sugar, granulated

- 1 tsp. of garlic, minced

- 1 tsp. of ginger, fresh, minced

- 1 x 14 & 1/4 oz. can of pureed tomatoes

Instructions:

1. Wash lentils in cool or cold tap water till it runs clear. Place lentils in pot with water sufficient to cover them.

2. Bring pot to boil. Cover. Reduce the heat down to med-low. Simmer and add water as needed while cooking, to keep the lentils covered till they are tender, or about 15-20 minutes. Drain the lentils.

3. Heat the oil in large-sized skillet on med. heat. Stir onions in and cook in oil till they caramelize, or about 18-20 minutes.

4. Mix the curry powder, curry paste, chili powder, cumin, turmeric, ginger, garlic, sugar and kosher salt in large sized bowl. Stir this into onions. Raise heat on stove top to high. Stir constantly while cooking till mixture is fragrant, usually just one or two minutes.

5. Add and stir tomato puree, then remove from the heat. Stir it into lentils and serve.

Nutrition Information

Serving size: 1 small bowl

Calories: 195

Fat: 2.5 grams

Carbohydrates: 33 grams

Protein: 12 grams

Cholesterol: 0 milligrams

Sodium: 569 milligrams

12 – Sesame Shrimp & Broccoli

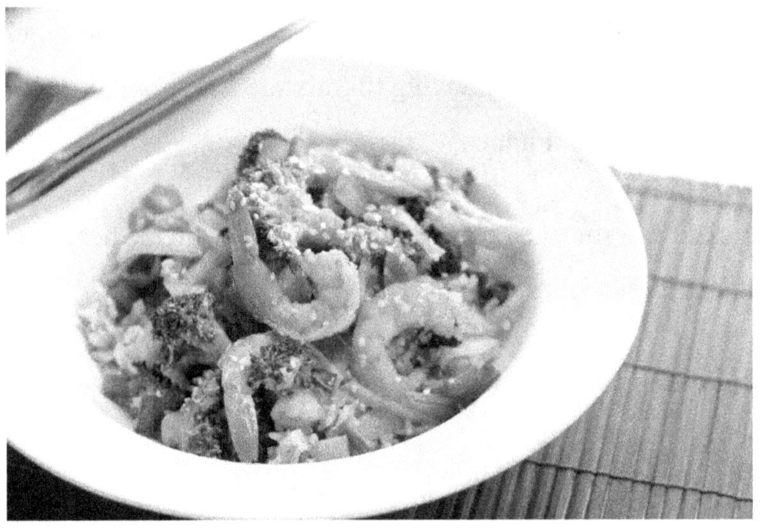

Sesame shrimp is normally fried & coated with a sweet and sticky sauce. In this recipe, sesame seeds are incorporated into a light panko coating. It has less sugar and more flavor than the original.

Makes 4 Servings

Cooking + Prep Time: 25 minutes

Ingredients:

- 1 & 1/2 tbsp. of sugar, brown
- 1 tbsp. of Sriracha sauce, bottled

- 2 whites from large eggs

- 1/2 cup of bread crumbs, whole wheat

- 1/4 cup of sesame seeds, toasted

- 1 & 1/2 lbs. of tail-intact, peeled, de-veined shrimp, large

- 2 tbsp. of oil, canola

- 1 tbsp. of sesame oil, toasted

- 1/2 tsp. of salt, kosher

- 1/2 tsp. of pepper, ground

- 1 tbsp. of garlic, sliced

- 1 tbsp. of peeled, chopped ginger, fresh

- 2 x 12-ounce broccoli heads with stems, cut in florets

- 1/4 cup of water, filtered

Instructions:

1. Whisk Sriracha sauce, egg whites and brown sugar together in shallow dish.

2. Combine sesame seeds and bread crumbs in separate shallow dish.

3. Work in batches to add the shrimp to the egg mixture and then dredge in the bread crumb mixture.

4. Heat 1 & 1/2 tsp. of sesame oil & 1 & 1/2 tsp. of canola oil in large skillet on med-high heat.

5. Add 1/2 of the dredged shrimp and cook till they are golden brown in color, or two to three minutes on each side. Remove them from the skillet. Repeat the procedure with the rest of the sesame and canola oils and remaining pre-dredged shrimp. Sprinkle the shrimp with 1/4 tsp. of kosher salt & 1/4 tsp. of ground pepper.

6. Heat last 1 tbsp. of canola oil in a pan on med-high heat. Add the ginger and garlic and stir constantly while cooking for one minute.

7. Add the broccoli and cook till browned lightly, two minutes or so. Add the filtered water. Cover the pan. Cook broccoli till crisp but tender, about two to three minutes. Remove cover from pan. Sprinkle with last 1/4 tsp. of kosher salt and last 1/4 tsp. of ground pepper. Serve broccoli with the shrimp.

Nutrition Information

Serving size: 8 shrimp + 1 cup of broccoli

Calories: 390

Fat: 18 grams

Protein: 35 grams

Carbohydrates: 26 grams

Sugars: 9 grams

Sodium: 679 milligrams

13 – Black Beans & Quinoa

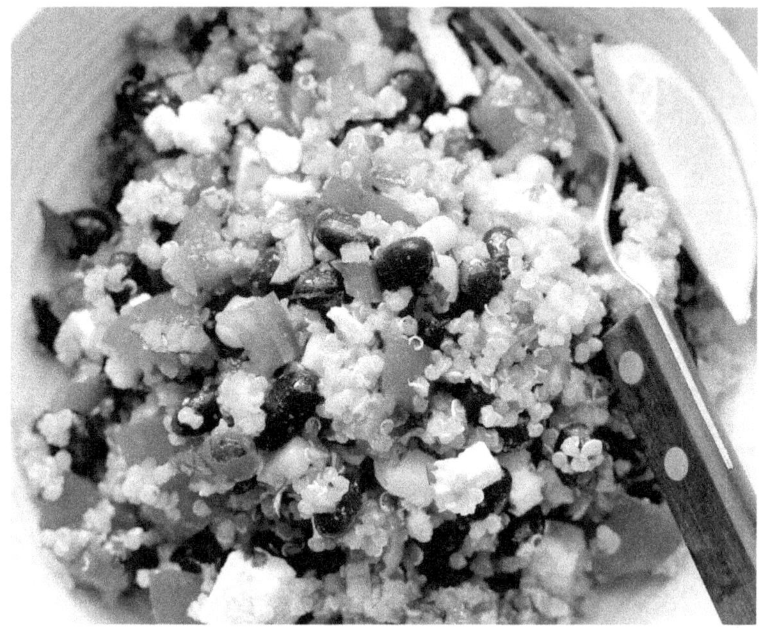

Using quinoa **Makes** this a tasty, slimming alternative to serving black beans with rice. Quinoa is a delicious and nutty grain that comes from South America.

Makes 10 Servings

Cooking + Prep Time: 55 minutes

Ingredients:

- 1 tsp. of oil, vegetable
- 1 chopped onion
- 3 chopped garlic cloves
- 3/4 cup of quinoa
- 1 & 1/2 cups of broth, vegetable
- 1/4 tsp. of pepper, cayenne
- 1 tsp. of cumin, ground
- Salt, kosher, as desired
- Pepper, ground, as desired
- 1 cup of corn kernels, frozen
- 2 x 15-oz. cans of rinsed, drained black beans
- 1/2 cup of chopped cilantro, fresh

Instructions:

1. Heat the oil in pan on med. heat. Stir while cooking the garlic and onion till browned lightly, or about eight to 10 minutes.

2. Add quinoa to mixture and mix well. Cover with broth. Season using cayenne pepper and cumin, then use kosher salt and ground pepper as desired.

3. Bring mixture to boil. Cover the pan. Reduce the heat, then summer till broth has been absorbed and the quinoa has become tender, usually 18-20 minutes or so.

4. Stir the corn into pan. Continue simmering till mixture has heated fully through, or about five minutes. Add and mix cilantro and black beans. Serve.

Nutrition Information

Serving size: 1 small bowl

Calories: 150

Fat: 2 grams

Carbohydrates: 28 grams

Protein: 7.5 grams

Cholesterol: 0 milligrams

Sodium: 510 grams

14 – Chicken with Farro

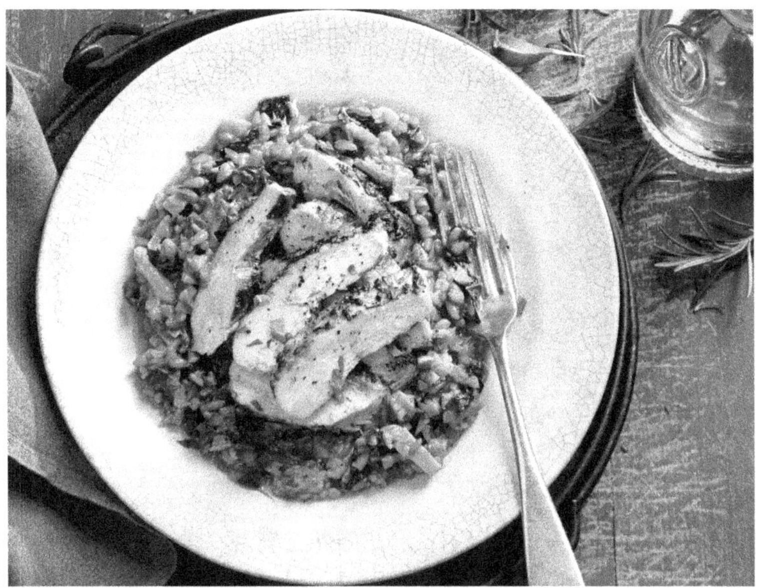

The chicken thighs in this recipe hold up well in your slow cooker. They surrender their rich juices, making the farro even more satisfying than it usually is.

Makes 4 Servings

Cooking + Prep Time: 25 minutes + 7 to 8 hours slow cooker time

Ingredients:

- 2 tbsp. of oil, olive
- 4 x 6-ounce chicken thighs, skin-on, bone-in
- 1/2 tsp. of salt, kosher
- 1/2 tsp. of pepper, black
- Non-stick spray
- 3 cups of chicken stock, unsalted
- 1 cup of farro, pearled, uncooked
- 1/2 cup of shallots, chopped
- 10 pitted, sliced olives, Castelvetrano
- 1 & 1/2 tbsp. of capers, drained
- 1/2 cup of chopped parsley, flat-leaf, fresh
- 1/4 cup of chopped almonds, toasted
- 1 tsp. of lemon zest, fresh
- 1 tbsp. of lemon juice, fresh
- 1 grated clove of garlic
- 1/4 tsp. of red pepper, crushed
- For garnishing: parsley leaves, flat-leaf, fresh

Instructions:

1. Heat the oil in large sized skillet on med-high heat.

2. Sprinkle the chicken using 1/4 tsp. of kosher salt & 1/4 tsp. of ground pepper.

3. Cook the chicken till it has browned, which takes two minutes or so on each side. Set the chicken aside.

4. Coat slow cooker with non-stick spray. Stir farro, stock, shallots, remaining kosher salt and remaining ground pepper together in the slow cooker.

5. Top the mixture with the reserved chicken. Sprinkle it with capers and olives. Cover the slow cooker. Cook on the low setting till inserted thermometer reads 165F, which takes seven to eight hours.

6. Remove the chicken from the slow cooker and add the almonds, parsley, lemon juice and zest, red pepper and garlic to the farro mixture. Then stir it till it has a creamy consistency. Use parsley leaves to garnish, then serve.

Nutrition Information

Serving size: 1 chicken thigh + 1 & 1/8 cups of farro

Calories: 515

Fat: 25 grams

Protein: 35 grams

Carbohydrates: 40 grams

Sugars: 4 grams

Sodium: 660 milligrams

15 – Braised Chicken

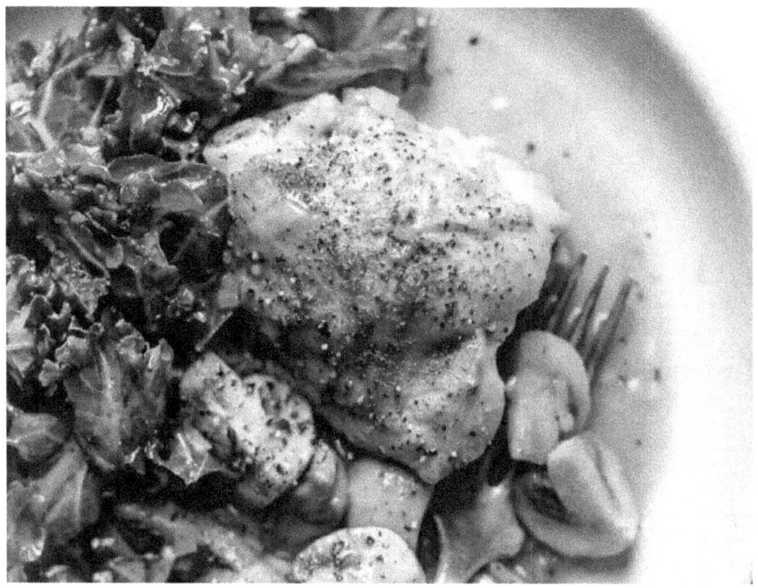

Braised chicken is so tasty with pasta or rice, and it's a great way to help you stay slim. Add some green beans to make it into a pleasing side dish.

Makes 6 Servings

Cooking + Prep Time: 40 minutes

Ingredients:

- 6 halved chicken breasts, boneless, skinless
- 1 tsp. of salt, garlic

- Black pepper, ground, as desired

- 2 tbsp. of oil, olive

- 1 sliced onion

- 1 x 14 & 1/2-oz. can of tomatoes, diced

- 1/2 cup of vinegar, balsamic

- 1 tsp. each of dried basil, oregano & rosemary

- 1/2 tsp. of thyme, dried

Instructions:

1. Season each side of the chicken breasts using garlic salt & ground pepper.

2. Heat the oil in large skillet on med. heat. Cook the seasoned chicken till it browns, about three or four minutes each side. Add the onion. Stir while cooking till the onion browns.

3. Pour the vinegar and tomatoes over the chicken. Season the mixture with oregano, basil, thyme and rosemary. Simmer till middle of chicken isn't pink anymore and the juices are running clear. This usually takes 15 minutes or so. Instant-read thermometer in center of chicken should read 165F or higher. Serve.

Nutrition Information

Serving size: 1 small plate

Calories: 198

Fat: 8 grams

Cholesterol: 60 milligrams

Sodium: 515 milligrams

Carbohydrates: 7.7 grams

Protein: 23.9 grams

16 – Quinoa & Tuna Toss

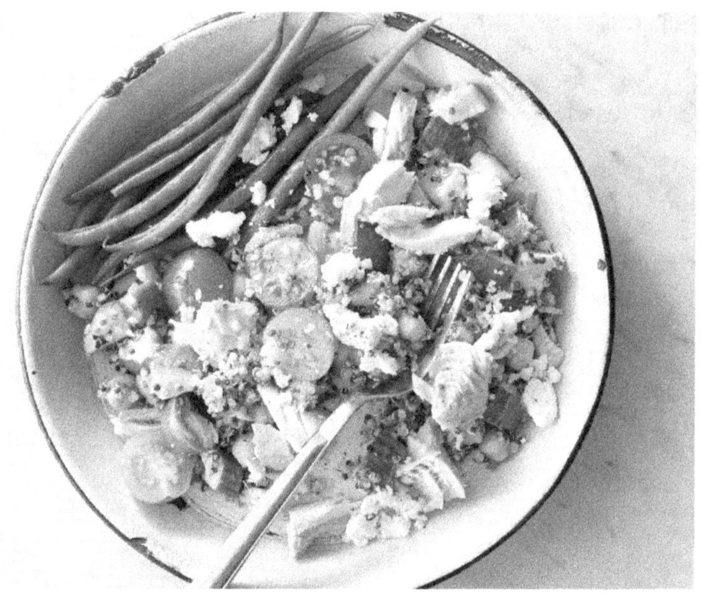

A protein bowl with its whole-grain goodness is a great solution when you need to throw together a quick lunch. You can cook the quinoa ahead of time, if you like.

Makes 1 Serving

Cooking + Prep Time: 15 minutes

Ingredients:

- 2 tsp. of oil, olive
- 1 tsp. of vinegar, red wine

- 1/2 tsp. of lemon juice, fresh

- 1/2 tsp. of mustard, Dijon

- 1 dash salt, kosher

- 1 dash pepper, ground

- 1/2 cup of quinoa, cooked

- 1/4 cup of rinsed, drained, canned chick peas, unsalted

- 1/4 cup of cucumber, chopped

- 1 tbsp. of feta cheese crumbles

- 5 halved cherry tomatoes

- 1 x 2.6-ounce packet of solid tuna, white, in water

Instructions:

1. Combine the first six ingredients in a bowl and stir well with whisk.

2. Combine quinoa and the rest of the ingredients in separate bowl.

3. Drizzle the mixture with dressing, gently tossing till ingredients are coated. Serve.

Nutrition Information

Serving size: 1 & 3/4 cup

Calories: 370

Fat: 15 grams

Protein: 29 grams

Carbohydrates: 30 grams

Cholesterol: 40 milligrams

Sodium: 455 milligrams

Sugars: 5 grams

17 – Pork Tenderloin with Tequila & Lime Sauce

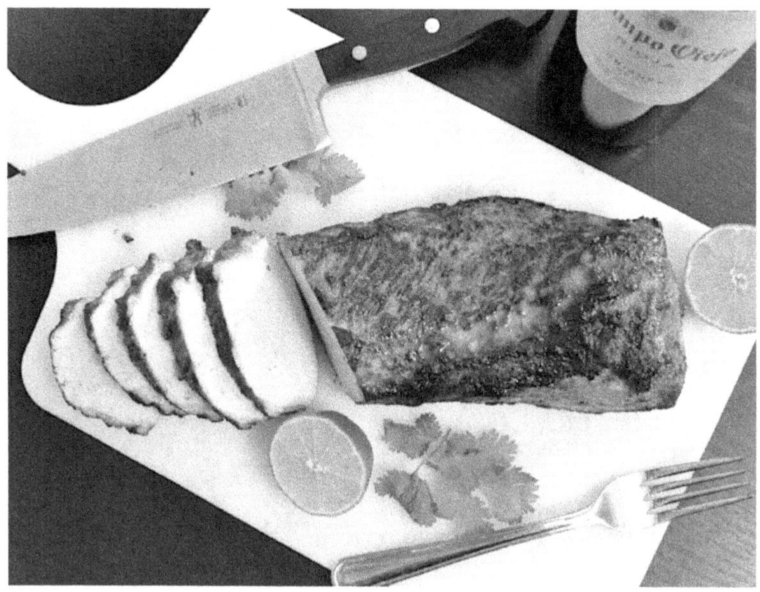

Marinating the pork overnight with this lovely marinade will give the meat a wonderful grilled lime flavor. You can freeze one tenderloin for a future slimming meal, too.

Makes 12 Servings

Cooking + Prep Time: 40 minutes + 8 hours marinating time

Ingredients:

- 1 cup of lime juice, fresh
- 1/2 cup of tequila
- 1/2 cup of orange juice, fresh
- 1/4 cup of chopped cilantro, fresh
- 2 tbsp. of chopped chilies, green
- 1 & 1/2 tbsp. of chili powder
- 1 tsp. of garlic, minced
- 1 tbsp. of honey, pure
- 1 tsp. of salt, kosher
- 3/4 tsp. of pepper, ground
- 2 med-sized pork tenderloins

Instructions:

1. Whisk orange juice, tequila, lime juice, chilies, cilantro, garlic, honey, chili powder, kosher salt & ground pepper in large-sized bowl. Pour into 1-gallon zipper top bag and add pork. Zip the bag closed and place in refrigerator for the overnight.

2. Preheat your outdoor grill on high. Oil grate lightly.

3. Combine marinade and pork. Cook meat on grill and turn them occasionally, till internal temperature of meat is 145F. This usually takes 18-20 minutes or so. Remove meat from grill and serve.

Nutrition Information

Serving Size: 1/12 recipe

Calories: 110

Fat: 2.5 grams

Carbohydrates: 5.5 grams

Protein: 12 grams

Cholesterol: 32 milligrams

Sodium: 231 milligrams

18 – Carrot & Tahini Soup

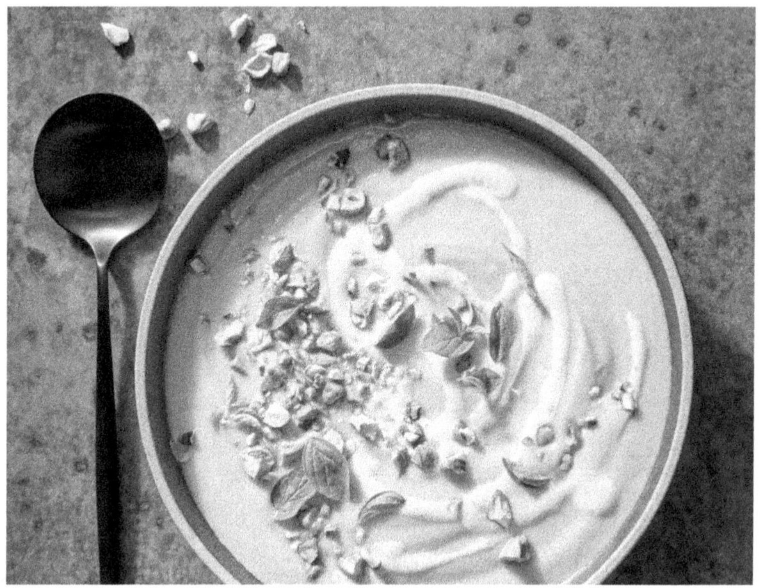

This recipe will allow you to enjoy a creamy, fresh-tasting soup without having to rely on butter or heavy cream for its flavor. The toasted sesame oil gives the soup depth.

Makes 4 Servings

Cooking + Prep Time: 40 minutes

Ingredients:

- 1 tbsp. of oil, olive
- 1 large chopped onion, yellow

- 1/2 tsp. of salt, kosher

- 1/2 tsp. of paprika, smoked

- 1/4 tsp. of turmeric, ground

- 2 chopped cloves of garlic

- 1 lb. of peeled, chopped carrots

- 3 cups of stock, unsalted vegetable or unsalted chicken

- 3 tbsp. of sesame seed paste

- 8 tsp. of tahini sauce, bottled

- 6 tbsp. of chopped pistachios, unsalted

- 2 tsp. of oregano leaves, fresh

Instructions:

1. Heat the oil in large sized Dutch oven on med-high heat. Add the onion and sauté for five to six minutes. Add and stir paprika, salt, garlic and turmeric and cook for one minute.

2. Add the carrots and cook for another minute. Add and stir stock and bring to boil. Reduce the heat down to med-low. Cover pot. Simmer for 18-20 minutes, till carrots have become quite tender.

3. Combine that carrot mixture with 3 tbsp. of sesame seed paste in blender. Remove the center portion of lid so steam

can escape and place lid on the blender. Place clean towel on lid opening so it won't splatter. Process carrot mixture till you have a smooth consistency.

4. Divide the soup evenly in four individual bowls. Drizzle 2 tsp. of tahini sauce on each. Top each bowl with 1/2 tsp. of oregano leaves and 1 & 1/2 tbsp. of pistachios. Serve.

Nutrition Information

Serving size: 1 & 1/4 cup

Calories: 280

Fat: 18 grams

Protein: 9 grams

Carbohydrates: 25 grams

Sodium: 459 milligrams

Sugars: 10 grams

19 – Potato Curry & Cauliflower

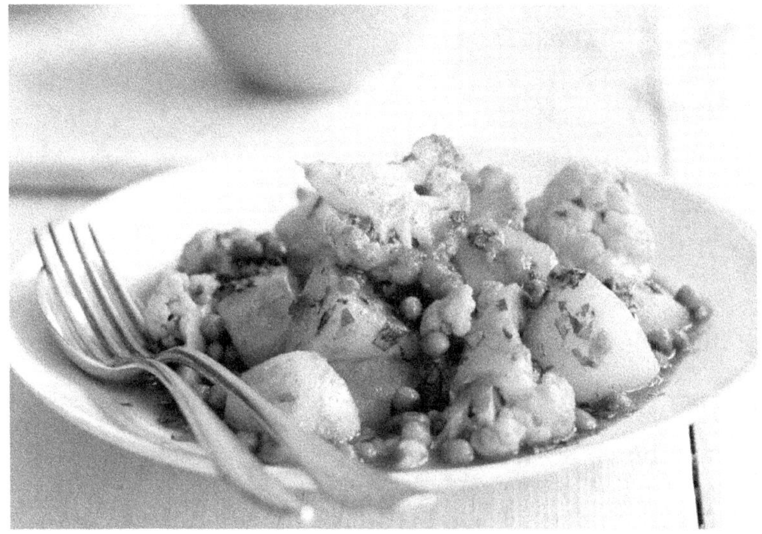

This is a traditional Indian curry and cauliflower dish that is filling, but still helps you to keep slim. You can add peas, too, if you like.

Makes 4 Servings

Cooking + Prep Time: 40 minutes

Ingredients:

- 1 floret-cut head of cauliflower
- 3 peeled, chunk-cut potatoes
- 1 tbsp. of oil, olive

- 1 tsp. of cumin seeds

- 1 chopped onion

- 2 diced tomatoes

- 1 tsp. of salt, kosher

- 1 tsp. of curry powder.

Instructions:

1. Place cauliflower florets in large glass dish. Cook on high in microwave for two or three minutes. Transfer florets to another bowl. Set it aside.

2. Place potatoes in a glass dish. Cook on high in microwave for four minutes. Pour potatoes into cauliflower bowl.

3. Heat oil and cumin seeds in large-sized skillet on med-high till the cumin has swelled and turned a golden brown in color. Add and stir onions into oil. Cook for three minutes or so.

4. Add tomatoes. Stir while cooking for three more minutes. Fold potatoes and cauliflower into mixture. Season using salt & curry powder. Continue to cook till mixture is fully heated, or three to five minutes. Serve while hot.

Nutrition Information

Serving size: 1 bowl

Calories: 230

Fat: 4 grams

Carbohydrates: 45 grams

Protein: 7.7 grams

Cholesterol: 0 milligrams

Sodium: 641 milligrams

20 – Arugula & Quinoa Bowl

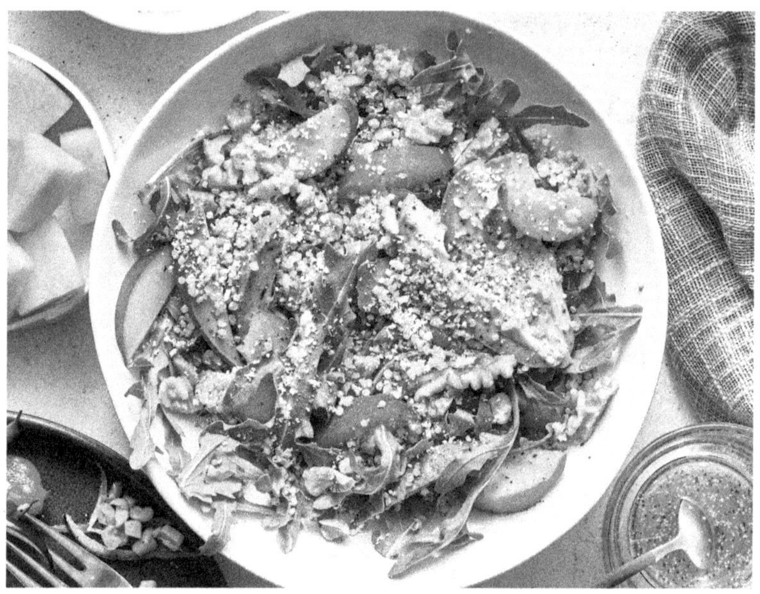

Here is a salad offering many textures and flavors, from quinoa and arugula to walnuts, cheese and peaches. It's easy to make and handy to take to carry-in dinners.

Makes 1 Serving

Cooking + Prep Time: 10 minutes

Ingredients:

- 1 tbsp. of vinegar, sherry
- 2 tsp. of oil, olive

- 1/8 tsp. of salt, kosher

- 1/8 tsp. of pepper, ground

- 1 cup of arugula greens

- 3/4 cup of quinoa, pre-cooked

- 1/2 sliced avocado

- 1/4 cup of peaches, chopped

- 2 tbsp. of walnuts, chopped

- 2 tsp. of Cotija or feta cheese crumbles

Instructions:

1. Whisk the oil, vinegar, kosher salt and ground pepper together in small sized bowl.

2. Place arugula in bottom of medium-sized bowl. Arrange quinoa, sliced avocado, walnuts and peaches around bowl's sides. Drizzle using vinaigrette. Sprinkle with the cheese crumbles and serve.

Nutrition Information

Serving size: 1 bowl

Calories: 550

Fat: 40 grams

Carbohydrates: 47 grams

Sugar: 7 grams

Sodium: 341 milligrams

21 – Tilapia with Mango Salsa

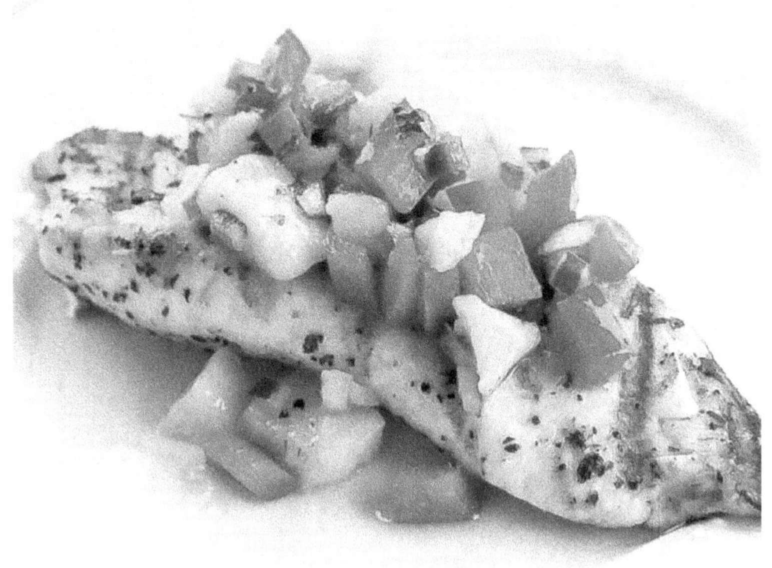

In this dish, tilapia is served with a wonderful fruit salsa. It can be served over chicken, as well. You'd never know it's geared for slimming menu plans, because it's so tasty.

Makes 4 Servings

Cooking + Prep Time: 45 minutes

Ingredients:

- 1/2 peeled, then cored & chopped pineapple, fresh
- 1/2 lb. of quartered strawberries

- 3 peeled, diced kiwi fruits

- 1 peeled, then de-seeded & diced mango, large

- 1/2 cup of tomatoes, grape

- 2 tbsp. of chopped cilantro, fresh

- 1 tbsp. of vinegar, balsamic

- 1 & 1/2 lbs. tilapia fillets

- 1/2 tsp. of pepper blend, seasoned

Instructions:

1. Toss vinegar, cilantro, tomatoes, mango, kiwi, strawberries and pineapple together in large sized bowl.

2. Spray large skillet using non-stick spray. Heat on med-high. Sprinkle the tilapia using the seasoned ground pepper blend. Fry in pan till fish is opaque and white, two to three minutes each side. Top the fish with fruit salsa and serve.

Nutrition Information

Serving size: 1/4 of recipe

Calories: 310

Fat: 3.2 grams

Carbohydrates: 35.5 grams

Protein: 37.1 grams

Cholesterol: 63 milligrams

Sodium: 84 milligrams

22 – Shaved Vegetable & Tuna Salad

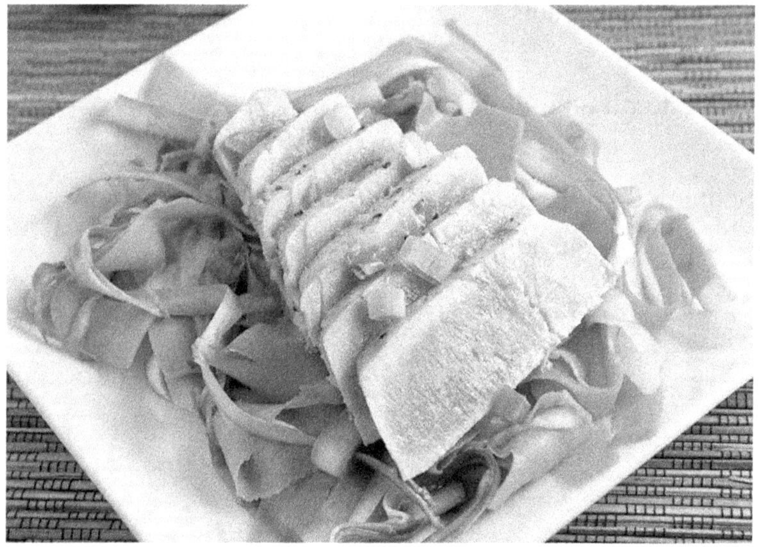

Veggies are very popular in the winter, and they can be roasted till they're tender. Shaving them into a salad as a side dish is a great alternative. They only take several minutes to make.

Makes 4 Servings

Cooking + Prep Time: 20 minutes

Ingredients:

- 1/4 cup of oil, olive
- 1 tbsp. of vinegar, rice

- 1 tsp. of salt, sea

- 3/4 tsp. of mustard, Dijon

- 3/4 tsp. of honey, pure

- 4 oz. of thinly shaved beets, baby gold

- 1 x 4-ounce trimmed, shaved bulb of fennel

- 4 oz. of shaved turnips, baby

- 1 x 6-ounce thinly sliced apple, Granny Smith

- 4 x 6-ounce tuna steaks

- 2 tsp. of sesame seeds, toasted

- 1/2 tsp. of pepper, ground

- 1 tbsp. of fennel fronds, torn

Instructions:

1. Combine vinegar, 2 tbsp. of oil, 1/2 tsp. of sea salt, honey and mustard in large sized bowl. Add the fennel, beets, apple and turnips. Coat by tossing. Sprinkle with the sesame seeds.

2. Heat the rest of the oil in skillet on high heat. Sprinkle the tuna using pepper & the last 1/2 tsp. of sea salt. Place them in hot pan. Cook for 90 seconds per side if you like your tuna rare, or till done as you desire.

3. Remove the tuna from the pan. Slice very thinly. Add to salad and top with the fronds of fennel. Serve.

Nutrition Information

Serving Size: 1 tuna steak + 1 & 1/4 cup of salad

Calories: 370

Fat: 16 grams

Protein: 44 grams

Carbohydrates: 13 grams

Cholesterol: 65 milligrams

Sodium: 640 milligrams

Sugars: 9 grams

23 – Marinated Cucumbers

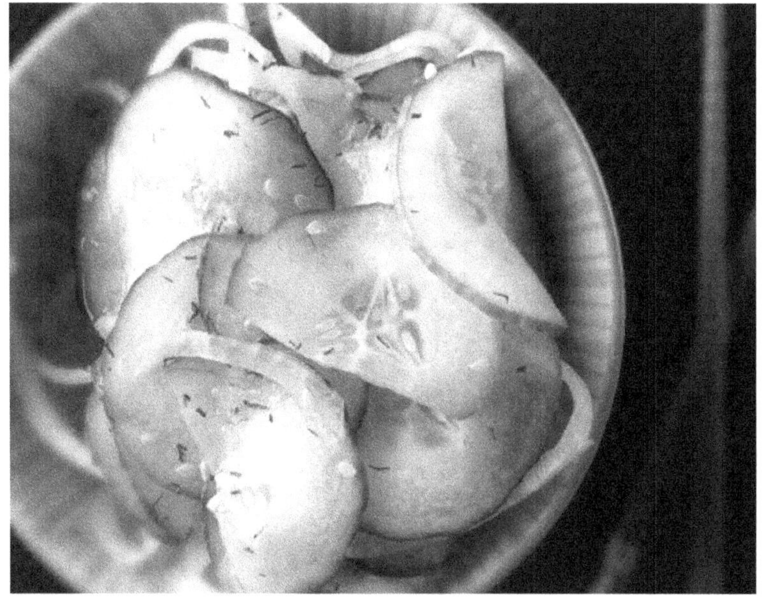

This recipe has been handed down through generations of healthy eaters. It tastes especially great in warmer months, and it's slim-recipe friendly.

Makes 4 Servings

Cooking + Prep Time: 15 minutes + 8 hours overnight setting time

Ingredients:

- 1/2 cup of sugar, granulated

- 1/2 cup of vinegar, white

- 1/2 tsp. of salt, kosher

- 1/4 tsp. of celery seed

- 1/4 cup of sliced onion, sweet

- 2 sliced cucumbers, medium or large

Instructions:

1. Whisk the sugar into the vinegar and add celery seed and kosher salt. Combine in large-sized bowl.

2. Add and stir in onions and cucumbers. Cover. Place in refrigerator overnight. Serve while cold.

Nutrition Information

Serving size: 1/4 of recipe

Calories: 116

Fat: 0.3 grams

Carbohydrates: 30 grams

Protein: 0.9 grams

Sodium: 295 milligrams

24 – Steak & Brussels Sprouts

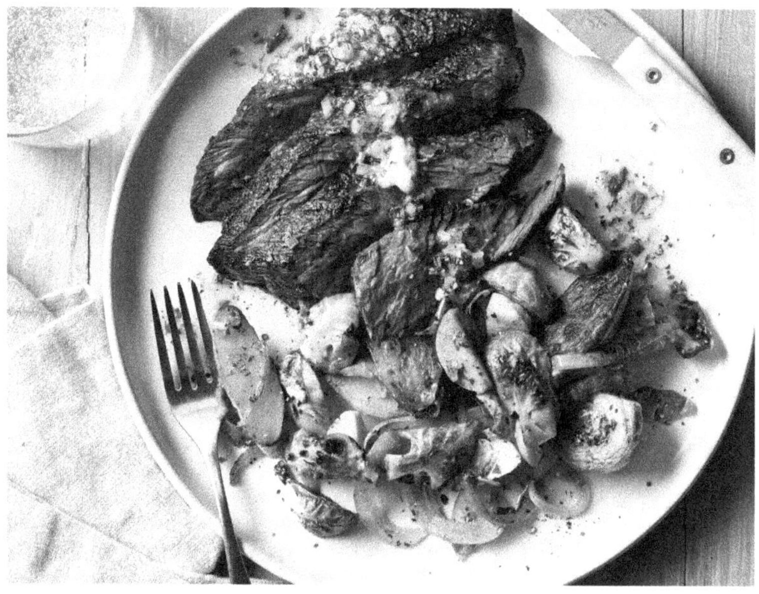

Steak & Brussels sprouts is a dish you can make in one pan and it's a very satisfying dinner. The steak is broiled directly over your vegetables, so the meat juices will baste them as they are caramelizing.

Makes 4 Servings

Cooking + Prep Time: 30 minutes

Ingredients:

- 6 oz. of trimmed, halved Brussels sprouts

- 6 oz. of halved, sliced sweet potatoes

- 2 tbsp. of oil, olive

- 1 x 1-pound trimmed steak, flat iron

- 2 tsp. of chopped thyme, fresh

- 1 tsp. of salt, kosher

- 3/4 tsp. of pepper, ground

Instructions:

1. Preheat the broiler with an oven rack six inches from the heat.

2. Place potatoes and Brussels sprouts on baking pan with rim. Toss with 1 tbsp. of oil. Spread out evenly in one layer. Place wire rack in the pan over the vegetables.

3. Rub the steak with 1 & 1/2 tsp. of oil. Place on the rack on top of veggies. Sprinkle the steak with 1 tsp. of thyme, 1/2 tsp. of kosher salt & 1/2 of ground pepper.

4. Broil steak and vegetables for 8-10 minutes. Turn the steak over and drizzle with the last 1 & 1/2 tsp. of oil. Sprinkle with last of thyme, kosher salt & ground pepper. Broil for five minutes, or till done as you desire.

5. Remove the steak from the pan. Allow to set for three to five minutes. Slice thinly, across the steak's grain. Place the veggies in medium bowl. Add pan juices. Toss and coat well. Serve.

Nutrition Information

Serving size: 3 ounces of steak + 1 cup of vegetables

Calories: 285

Fat: 16 grams

Protein: 25 grams

Carbohydrates: 12 grams

Cholesterol: 40 milligrams

Sodium: 570 milligrams

Sugars: 4 grams

25 – Middle Eastern Salad

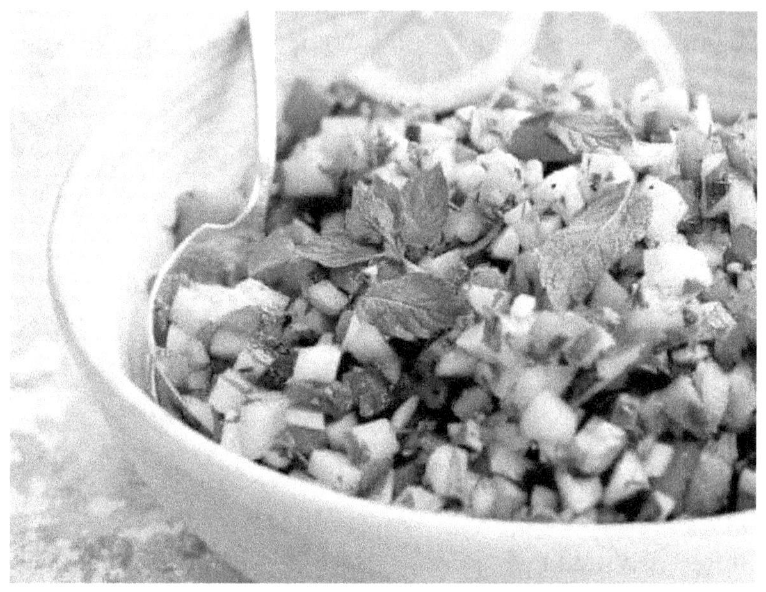

This slim diet-friendly dish transforms brown rice into a Middle-Eastern delight, when you add dates, cumin, mint and chick peas. The dates offer fiber, which helps to suppress appetite.

Makes 4 Servings

Cooking + Prep Time: 25 minutes

Ingredients:

- 2 tbsp. of oil, olive
- 1/2 sliced onion, sweet
- 1 x 16-oz. can of rinsed, drained chick peas
- 1/2 tsp. of cumin, ground
- 1/4 tsp. of salt, kosher
- Pepper, ground
- 3 cups of brown rice, cooked
- 1/2 cup of dates, pitted and chopped
- 1/4 cup of fresh mint, chopped
- 1/4 cup of parsley, fresh

Instructions:

1. Heat the oil in large skillet on med-high. Add the onion. Stir often while cooking till onion has begun to brown. Remove from the heat. Add and stir chick peas, ground cumin and kosher salt. Season as desired with ground pepper.

2. Combine the chick pea/onion mixture with rice, mint, parsley and dates in large sized bowl. Toss till combined thoroughly. Serve while warm.

Nutrition Information

Serving size: 1 bowl

Calories: 395

Fat: 10 grams

Saturated Fat: 1 gram

Protein: 7 grams

Carbohydrates: 67 grams

Sodium: 355 milligrams

Who says you can't have dessert when you're eating healthy? These recipes are delicious, decadent and they'll still help you slim down or remain slim…

26 – Healthy Fruit Salad

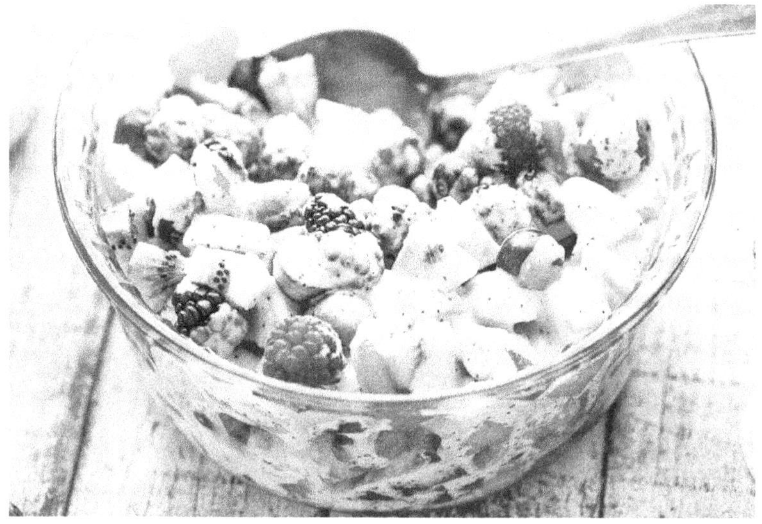

This is a family favorite recipe, and easy to make when company shows up without calling ahead. You can swap lemon yogurt for strawberry, if you like.

Makes 12 Servings

Cooking + Prep Time: 15 minutes

Ingredients:

- 1 pint of sliced strawberries, fresh
- 1 lb. of halved green grapes, seedless
- 3 peeled, sliced bananas

- 1 x 8-oz. container of yogurt, strawberry

Instructions:

1. Toss yogurt, bananas, grapes and strawberries together in large sized bowl. Serve promptly.

Nutrition Information

Serving size: 1/12 of recipe

Calories: 84

Fat: 1/2 gram

Protein: 1 & 1/2 grams

Sodium: 12 grams

27 – Pomegranate & Vanilla Parfaits

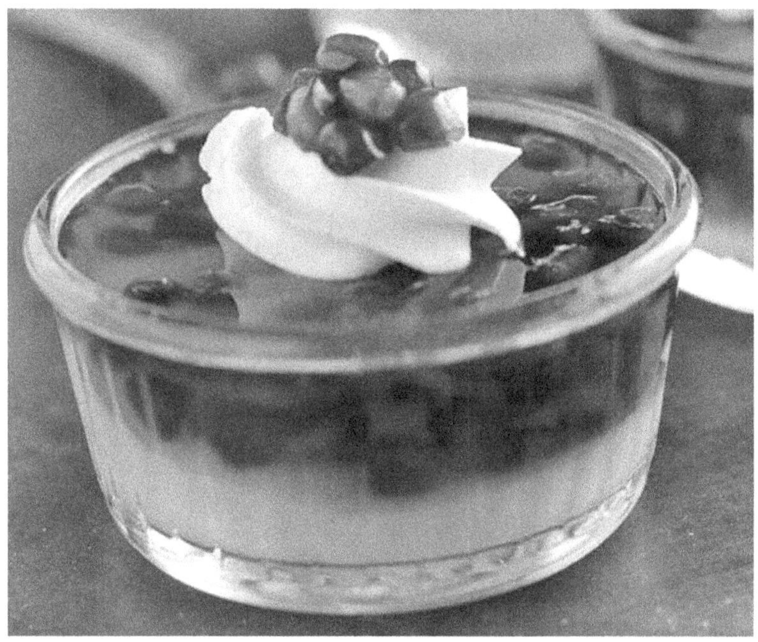

This creamy, rich pudding tempers the pomegranate's sweet-tart taste. Choose small bowls or dessert dishes for this delectable parfait.

Makes 6 Servings

Cooking + Prep Time: 3 hours & 55 minutes

Ingredients:

Pomegranate Compote

- 2 tbsp. o sugar, granulated
- 2 tsp. of corn starch
- 1 cup of pomegranate seeds
- 2/3 cup of pomegranate juice
- 1 tbsp. of lemon juice, fresh

Pudding

- 1 cup of milk, low-fat
- 3/4 cup of half-n-half
- 2 tsp. of vanilla extract, pure
- 1 egg, large
- 1 yolk from large egg
- 1/3 cup of sugar, granulated
- 1 & 1/2 tbsp. of corn starch
- 1 tbsp. of butter, unsalted

To garnish:

- 1/2 cup of pomegranate seeds
- 6 sprigs of mint

Instructions:

1. Mix 2 tsp. of corn starch with 2 tbsp. of sugar in small-sized sauce pan.

2. Add pomegranate juice and seeds and then lemon juice and combine by stirring.

3. Bring to boil on med-high. Stir while cooking for four or five minutes till mixture is syrupy. Transfer it to small sized bowl. Place in refrigerator.

4. Combine milk with half-n-half in heavy, medium-sized pan. Add the vanilla extract. Bring to simmer on med. heat. Remove from heat. Cover pan. Allow the mixture to steep for four to five minutes.

5. Whisk the egg yolk, egg, 1 & 1/2 tbsp. of corn starch and 1/3 cup of sugar in medium sized bowl.

6. Reheat milk mixture till barely steaming. Whisk 1/3 of steaming milk carefully into egg mixture. Pour the new mixture into same pan. Cook on med., and whisk constantly, till mixture is very thick, which usually takes two or three minutes. Remove the pan from heat. Add and whisk butter in.

7. Divide pomegranate compote in six x 3/4-cup ramekins. Spoon pudding mixture on top of compote. Cover. Refrigerate till pudding is firm and chilled well, which takes three hours or longer.

8. Garnish parfaits with mint and pomegranate seeds and serve.

Nutrition Information

Serving size: 1 parfait

Calories: 215

Fat: 9 grams

Saturated fat: 4 grams

Carbohydrates: 31 grams

Protein: 4 grams

Sugar: 28 grams

Sodium: 48 milligrams

28 – Berry Crisp Dessert

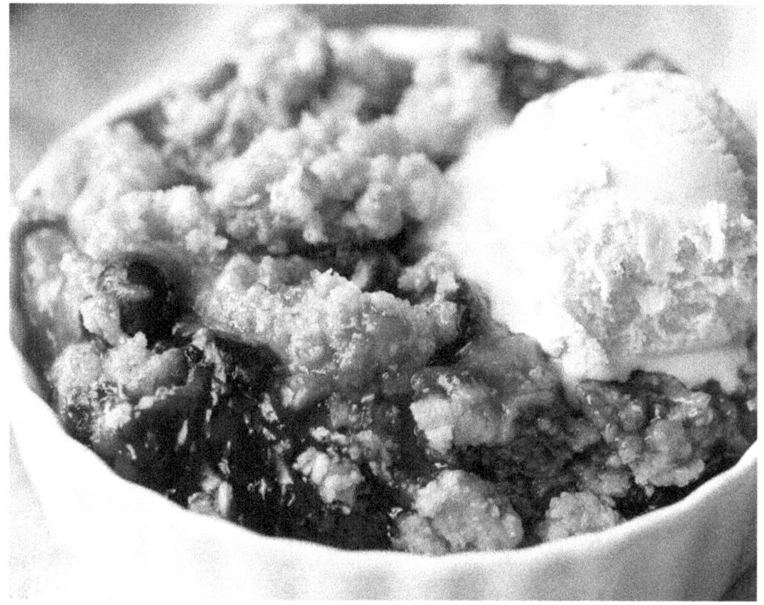

Do you have lots of berries from your garden or the local market in the summer months? Here's a great way to use them!

Makes 18 Servings

Cooking + Prep Time: 30 minutes

Ingredients:

- 2 cups of apples, sliced thinly
- 1 cup each of fresh blueberries, raspberries and blackberries
- 1 cup of rhubarb, chopped
- 3 tbsp. of corn starch
- 2 cups of sugar, granulated
- 1 tsp. of cinnamon, ground
- 1 pinch of nutmeg, ground
- 2 cups of oats, rolled
- 1 cup of sugar, brown, packed
- 1/2 cup of flour, all-purpose
- 1/4 cup of butter, unsalted
- 1/2 tsp. of cinnamon, ground

Instructions:

1. Preheat the oven to 400F.

2. Mix apples, all berries and rhubarb together in large sized bowl.

3. In separate bowl, combine corn starch, sugar, nutmeg and cinnamon together. Blend it with fruit mixture.

4. Pour the resulting mixture in 13" x 9" glass casserole dish.

5. To prepare topping, mix flour, oatmeal, 1/2 tsp. of cinnamon and brown sugar together in large sized bowl. Add butter in small sized pats. Cut into flour mixture till it is crumbly, but without any large chunks. Sprinkle topping over fruit.

6. Bake in 400F oven for 30-35 minutes, till topping has turned brown. Serve hot.

Nutrition Information

Serving size: 1/18 of recipe

Calories: 230

Fat: 3 grams

Carbohydrates: 48 grams

Protein: 2 grams

Sodium: 23 milligrams

29 – Pumpkin Pie

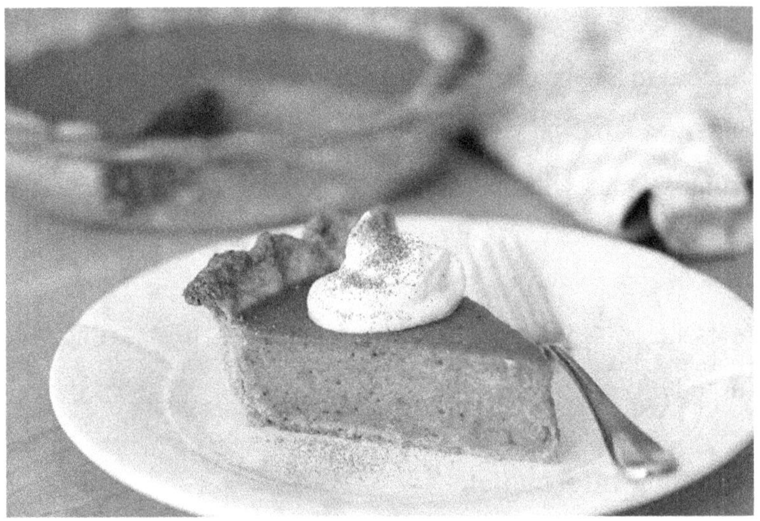

This pumpkin pie is sugar free and low carb, so it's perfect for a diet geared to slimming down. You'll never tell by tasting that it's gluten free, either.

Makes 10 Servings

Cooking + Prep Time: 1 & 1/4 hour

Ingredients:

- 1 x 15-ounce can of pureed pumpkin
- 1/2 cup of coconut milk, canned
- 1/2 cup of monk fruit

- 1 tsp. of cinnamon, ground

- 2 eggs, large

- 3/4 tsp. of ginger, ground

- 1/2 tsp. of nutmeg, ground

- 1/4 tsp. of cloves, ground

- 1 store-bought pie crust, low carb, cooled

Instructions:

1. Preheat oven to 350F.

2. Whisk all ingredients together in large sized bowl. Pour into pie crust.

3. Tent pie lightly using foil, so crust won't brown as much. Place in oven. Bake till center has a bit of a jiggle. Knife inserted near crust should come back clean. This usually takes between 45 and 50 minutes.

4. Turn oven off and crack oven door open a bit. Allow pie to sit in the oven for 1/2 hour.

5. After 1/2 hour, allow pie to sit on counter and cool FULLY for two hours. Then place in refrigerator for an hour or more. Serve.

Nutrition Information

Serving size: 1 slice, 1/10 of pie

Calories 204

Fat: 15 grams

Saturated Fat: 7 grams

Sodium: 202 milligrams

Carbohydrates: 13 grams

Fiber: 3 grams

Sugar: 2 grams

30 – Healthy Rice Pudding

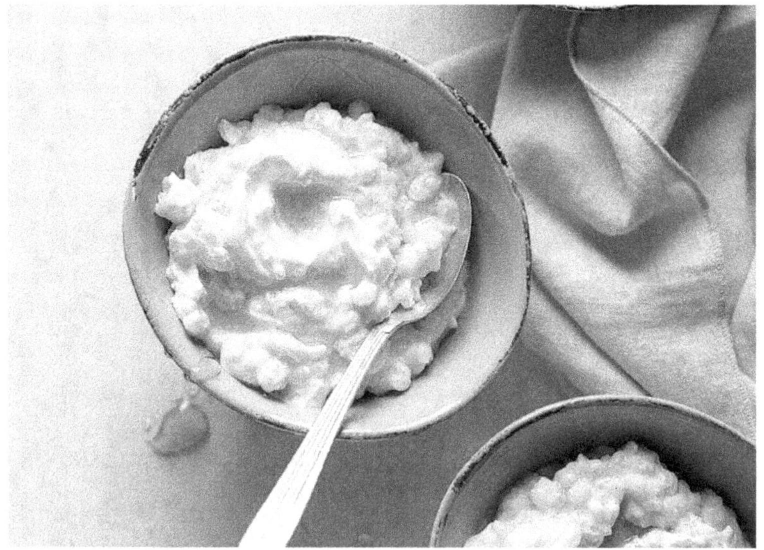

The secret to this healthier rice pudding is using brown rice, rather than white. With its raisins and vanilla, you'll find it nutritious as well as delicious.

Makes 4 Servings

Cooking + Prep Time: 1 hour & 10 minutes

Ingredients:

- 1 & 1/2 cups of water, filtered

- 3/4 cup of brown rice, uncooked

- 1 & 1/2 cups of milk, low-fat

- 1/3 cup of sugar, granulated

- 1/4 tsp. of salt, kosher

- 1/2 cup of milk, low-fat

- 1 beaten egg, large

- 2/3 cup of raisins

- 1 tbsp. of butter, unsalted

- 1/2 tsp. of vanilla extract, pure

Instructions:

1. Add rice to water in sauce pan on high heat. Bring to boil. Reduce the heat down to med-low. Cover pan. Simmer till rice becomes tender, usually 40-45 minutes.

2. In another pan, combine the 1 & 1/2 cups of milk with cooked rice, salt and sugar. Cook on med. heat till creamy and thick, which takes 15-20 minutes. Add and stir last 1/2 cup of milk, raisins and the beaten egg. Stir constantly while cooking for a couple minutes longer.

3. Remove pan from heat. Add and stir vanilla and butter. Serve while warm.

Nutrition Information

Serving size: 1/4 of recipe

Calories: 371

Fat: 6 & 1/2 grams

Saturated Fat: 3 grams

Sodium: 255 milligrams

Total Carbohydrates: 70 grams

Protein: 9 grams

Sugars: 35 grams

Conclusion

This slim recipe cookbook has shown you…

How to use different ingredients to affect unique tastes in healthy dishes both well-known and rare.

How can you include slim recipes in your home cooking?

You can…

- Make sweet and savory breakfasts like oatmeal and breakfast quiche, which I imagine everyone knows about. They are just as tasty as you have heard.
- Learn to cook with sweet potatoes and squash, which are widely used in slim recipes. Find them in the produce section of your local grocery store or farmer's market.
- Enjoy making delectable slim seafood dishes, including tuna and tilapia. Fish is a mainstay in healthy recipes, and there are SO many ways to make it great.
- Make dishes using broccoli and carrots, which are often used in weight loss recipes.

- Make various types of healthy desserts like pumpkin pie and pomegranate & vanilla parfaits that will tempt your family's sweet tooth.

Have fun experimenting! Enjoy the results!

www.ingramcontent.com/pod-product-compliance
Lightning Source LLC
Chambersburg PA
CBHW061720250726
48657CB00002B/691